Slow Cooker VS Pressure Cooker: Discover Pros and Cons of Healthy Eating Tools

Table of content

Introduction

It's time to take control of the parts of our lives that we can control. Is is possible to fit more hours into a day? Can we squeeze in 30 more minutes of workout time? What part of our lives is most controllable? Now is the time to find solutions for getting more nutrition, eating healthier, and feeling better about the food choices we make.

Nutritionists will tell you raw food is generally the best way to eat. The blender has become a go-to appliance in our kitchens as a way to convert raw fruits and vegetables into a quick, vitamin and mineral packed meal. But how many smoothies can one slurp before one gets heartily sick of green drinks, and longs for a meal or two that has some substance; a meal one can sink your teeth into.

You can prepare fresh fruits, vegetables, eggs, poultry, fish and meat in alternate ways. The slow cooker (crock pot) and the pressure cooker are two kitchen appliances/tools no one should be without. If you haven't used either the crock pot or the pressure cooker, read on! This book gives the reader additional choices to the blender as a way of preparing meals in the home.

Chapter 1 – Fresh is Better

It is very popular to throw some yoghurt along with lettuce, kale, cabbage, beets, strawberries, watermelon, cantaloupe, carrots, radishes, blueberries, all kinds of squash, pineapple, apples, and any other fruit or veggie in your fridge into a blender, hit the "frappe" button for 20 seconds and pour the concoction into a travel mug to hit the door with a smoothie in hand. It makes for a nutritious meal in very little time.

But let's face it, how many meals can you be happy slurping? Even if you vary the ingredients, you're still drinking your meal. Smoothies are good for you, but are they good for the soul? Do they satisfy our natural urge to munch, to chew?

How many meals can you make in a blender until your finer sensibilities revolt, and demand some REAL food?

If you're in a hurry for a meal, there's always fast food. You don't even need to leave your car. Just drive through, place your order, get your over-cooked, over salted, fried in grease wrapped in paper tasteless meal. What kind of nutritional value do you find in fast food? On the way home from a long day, are you too hungry to endure the thought of cooking? Does the idea of a thick green soup of a smoothie seem unappealing?

What if you could have fresh food made at home in a relatively short period of time? What if the food was waiting on you when you got home, already cooked and filling your place with enticing aromas? These two choices can be had with two great kitchen appliances/devices—the slow cooker (crock pot) and the pressure cooker.

The benefits of fresh food are virtually limitless. The food itself tastes better after you give your body some time to adjust to your new diet of fresh supple foods, and they also have ample nutritious benefits when compared to typical factory processed chemical-soaked products that you can buy in the super-store. So whether you choose to go with a pressure cooker or a crock pot, you can surely enjoy being able to reap the benefits of eating the typical ingredients that go into a crock pot or pressure cooker. They really are superior foods in every sense of the word.

The kinds of foods that go into crock pots or pressure cookers are typically vegetables and leaner meats if you happen to eat meat-- and the taste and flavors that come out of these ingredients when being cooked in these manners are just amazing for your pallet to experience. So either way, you will be having fresher, more natural foods-- and that's always a good thing.

Now that being said there are some differences between pressure cookers and crock pots. Crock pots take much longer to cook foods and will thus tend to blend flavors together in a soup-like texture. This is distinct from the individually-cooked elements of the pressure cooker.

The pressure cooker is much less blended, and more traditionally cooked-- though it's more or less a better option than other methods of cooking since it locks in the nutrients of the food without heating them and boiling them away in a grease or the open air that a pan will provide for the food.

There are other key pros and cons for both pressure cookers and crock pots, but the general benefit that they both share is that you're definitely going to be cooking with healthier ingredients that have improved taste and more culinary options than a blender will give you.

You're going to have the added benefits of making a vegetarian diet much more palatable and tasty for you, and you're also going to be able to manage your cooking with either implement much more easily.

What can we say? Fresh really is better. In all respects.

Chapter 2 – Arguments for the pressure cooker

There are some compelling reasons to go with the pressure cooker over the crock pot. For one, if you're a vegetarian, you're going to be able to have much more options with the pressure cooker than you will with the crock pot.

The crock pot tends to make vegetables seem all mushy and soupy whereas the pressure cooker still locks in and keeps all the high temperatures that cooking really needs to be effective in the first place and prepare your food in a way that's easier for your body to digest and your mouth to... well.. chew and process.

This can be hard for people who are vegetarians and want to find a few different options to cook with that will leave them more fulfilled than a smoothie or some other cheaply thrown-together belly-filling meal that really doesn't satisfy the pallet.

In contrast, a pressure cooker will have all kinds of benefits when cooking with vegetables. For instance, beans will be less mushy and more distinct for one to enjoy their true flavor. You can cook rice in a pressure cooker for that Japanese or otherwise referred to as 'sticky rice' effect that some people truly enjoy. The bottom line is the the distinct flavors that the pressure cooker allows when cooking vegetables also allows all kinds of other options that the slow cooker won't actually give you in the first place.

Beans are great in a pressure cooker because the pressure cooker cooks them so fast without having the beans split. This preserves the flavor and gives a whole different experience as well as a lot of different angles that you can cook from when it comes to food preparation involving beans or other well known protein sources from vegetables.

You'll be able to enjoy more variety with purely vegetarian dishes. That's one clear advantage that the pressure cooker has over the slow cooker.

That being said, that doesn't necessarily mean that you'll be limited to only vegetarian dishes with the pressure cooker. The pressure cooker can cook meats beautifully as well-- and will have as many versatile ways of cooking with the same nutrient-locking qualities that it always does. It really does depend on what you eat, but that is one clear advantage to the pressure cooker.

Another really good advantage that the pressure cooker has is the fact that it doesn't take up as much space in your kitchen practically speaking. The pressure cooker itself doubles as a very large pot/vat that you can use for other reasons. There is a locking lid that allows it to cook at very very high temperatures and significant pressures that gives it a unique preparation style that is out of this world when it comes to retaining nutrients.

But the real beauty of it is that it's very versatile and store-able, so if you have a kitchen with limited space, you're in luck if you've picked a pressure cooker over a slow cooker.

Just store and use the pot, and the lid itself can be easily hidden away for just when you want to use the pot as a pressure cooker. The point of this way of cooking is practicality and efficiency. And pressure cookers are efficient in just about every possible way. They're efficient with food-time preparation, they're efficient with storage space, and they're efficient again with locking in the natural nutrients that are normally cooked away with your normal food preparation methods.

However that's still not it when arguing for the pressure cooker over the slow cooker.

The major advantage is actually the time and stress that it takes to prepare the meal all together. If you're reading this, you probably cook for more than just one; you probably cook for other people as well. So you know the hassle that's involved with having to plan a whole day in advance what's going to be for dinner in the future.

That's something that all of us probably have in common when it comes to home preparation and home planning-- but how would you like to be able to just improvise a fantastic and nutritious meal in just an hour?

That right there is the major advantage that a pressure cooker has over a slow cooker; one is fast and the other is... well... slow. So with a pressure cooker you can just throw in just about any form of *"ingredients"* and in thirty minutes you'll have something that's at least vaguely edible regardless of how crazy your combination was in the beginning.

That's the worst scenario though; most of us are really good at improvising and picking ingredients that make sense together. That's the real power of pressure-cooking; the versatility of it all-- and the results that you get after the fact. That's what you really want is the efficient process of being able to make a good meal from home on the fly with what you probably already had without the stress of having to plan specific recipes.

Pressure cookers can cook meals in under thirty minutes. Slow cookers cannot. Case and point.

But actually, the benefits *still* don't actually end there. There are still more to come.

For example, some of the time you may find yourself at high altitude. Do you know how much the altitude can affect the quality of the food you prepare? Not with a pressure cooker! Pressure cookers have constant and consistent pressures that build up within them regardless of what altitude you happen to be cooking in.

So even if you live in like the Himalayan mountains, you can always rely on your pressure cooker to deliver a tasty and right-on-the-mark meal that's consistent with the recipe. No funny business that you get from altitudes messing with your food prep.

Altitude can and does affect how food cooks. Everything else practically besides the pressure cooker is affected by this. Baking, pan-searing, and yes, slow-cooking. The reason why these other methods are so susceptible to altitude is because at higher altitudes, the air gets thinner.

Thinner air is less dense-- so even when it is at the proper temperature to cook food, the food will still take significantly longer to cook due to the thinner air and thus worse method of delivering heat-energy to the food that you're trying to cook.

Pressure cookers lock the pressure inside the pot, so it contains much more of the thermal energy than, say, a pan would. A pan would radiate that heat out a lot more than a pressure cooker would. The pressure cooker is... again... much more efficient at storing and transferring heat-energy into foods and thus cooking them.

Chapter 3 – Argument for the slow cooker

Do you like spending effort that you don't have to? No. You probably don't.

That's exactly where the slow cooker comes in. The slow cooker is very lazy-friendly. It's a "whatever" cooking implement. The slow cooker brings a host of utterly unique recipes right to you with minimal effort and maximal taste. That's the way the slow cooker works.

What the slow cooker does is essentially cooks things very slowly at low temperatures to gently and gradually extrude the juices, flavors, and aromas of food into a broth or soup for you to enjoy. The slow cooker has a tendency to bring foods into an even consistency with a host of complex flavors blended beautifully and elegantly together. No other way of cooking can actually achieve what a slow cooker does.

So why is a slow cooker better than a pressure cooker?

For one-- it's less effort. Yes, it is technically more *time* to cook with a slow cooker, but slow cookers are much, much more forgiving than pressure cookers are. With a pressure cooker, if you over-salt or season a dish, then you've pretty much ruined the whole thing. With a slow cooker, you can just add a starch or something to balance out the saltiness-- you can play with it. You can, in a sense, 'make right' where pressure cookers are much more unforgiving.

With slow cookers you've got all the time in the world to actually prepare your meal. In the morning, you can throw some onions, chicken broth, beans, carrots, and just generally *whatever you like eating* in the crock pot, put it on medium heat, and then leave for the day.

When you come home, you'll have a meal that's more or less ready to plate and serve. So, yes, in a sense it takes more time for you to cook that-- but you're not really *spending* that time cooking your meal; it's all hands-off for the most part.

You can season with a slow cooker in ways that you really can't with a pressure cooker. Seasoning in a slow cooker is easier because slow cookers blend together spices and flavors in ways that no other way of cooking will actually be able to accomplish-- even blenders don't 'blend' as well as pressure cookers do. Believe it or not-- well... In a sense.

This blend of flavors is a really unique and good thing that you can only really accomplish with a slow cooker. Hummus, for example, is made with a slow cooker-- and pretty much you'll be able to find all kinds of recipes that call for a slow cooker exclusively. So if you like those foods, you'll pretty much have to use a slow cooker to get those things made and ready to go get plated and enjoyed by hungry people.

This also means that slow-cookers are really good at planning out meals for a long, long time. If you're the kind of person that likes to calculate and plan out your meals, then a slow cooker might be the best choice for you. It basically makes food taste really well, and cost relatively no effort whatsoever.

Honestly, the hardest thing about slow cooking is cleaning the slow cooker after you're done using it. That's honestly it.

But that's not all of the advantages that a slow cooker has over a pressure cooker.

While... yes... there are differences between a pressure cooker and a slow cooker; *most* of the things you can cook with a pressure cooker you can also cook with a slow cooker. So if you're going for what cooking instrument gives you the most range of foods you can prepare-- it's really the slow cooker.

The pressure cooker can give you the most variety in textures and flavors. It gives you more options in preparing the same dish in different ways. The slow cooker gives you much more dishes that you can prepare that will all taste great.

Another good thing that a slow cooker has that the pressure cooker doesn't is the fact that there's no wrong way to cook with a slow cooker. It's mostly identical. So you can actually claim that you're no better or worse than, say, Gordon Ramsey when it comes to slow cooking-- because for those six or eight hours when the slow cooker is brewing, the process is the same, regardless of what cook is standing over it.

Do you see now how forgiving slow cookers are? They're truly more efficient than the pressure cooker when it comes to efficiency of the effort and stress that you have to invest in bringing a meal to the table.

True, the slow cooker will have a tendency to make foods much more smoothly blended and more of a homogenous mixture than, say, the pressure cooker will. But that's... actually a good thing... depending on who you are and what you like.

Vegetables in slow cookers will tend to absorb more flavors from spices and stocks-- so that makes them much easier to eat. Think of slow cookers as being much better for people who are *trying* to be vegetarians. It makes vegetables much more palatable and less vegetable-tasting, while it still retains all the nutrients the vegetable provides.

This means that peas and cabbage and vinegars-- all those combinations of just regular stuff that you really wouldn't independently want to consume-- can all of a sudden (well... not really 'all of a sudden'-- but you get the picture) be blended together in a dish that's aromatically and texturally pleasing. It's amazing what slow cookers can do to making food more tasty. You can make boring foods much more wholesome and satisfying with a slow cooker as opposed to a pressure cooker.

Slow cookers are slower when it comes to actually cooking the food. That's probably why they're called a slow cooker. But that's something that most people will actually want. It's basically a pot that you can throw virtually any combination of ingredients in and make amazing dishes out of hours later without you having to put any specific effort into it. It's just... convenient like that.

You can do chicken and dumplings and just all kinds of stuff in a slow cooker. It's really fantastic for soups as well, and again it's good for getting the full flavor of anything to actually reach your taste buds. The smooth textures that slow cookers tend to produce are an added benefit as well. So you can really do about the same thing with just about an endless variety of base ingredients.

Slow cookers produce really, really good food-- pretty much regardless of what you put in there as long as what you put in there is vaguely edible to begin with. Heck-- you can even cook peas with nuts and get the flavor of a nut cooked into the peas when you eat them.

This is particularly good for stews that have a bit of meat in them but lots of vegetables. This is great if you're trying to lose weight and develop a taste for vegetables but you're not quite at the spot where you can give up meat entirely cold turkey. This way, you can have a diet that's 80% vegetarian without actually having to feel that you're missing out on having meats at all. That's a huge benefit to slow cooking.

So in summary, slow cookers are just really fantastically convenient to use because you only have to invest like... ten or so actual minutes that you have to spend really preparing the dish. That's crazy. You can literally spend like two minutes just picking ingredients from your kitchen, then you can throw them all into a pot with water, set the thing to cook, then *go take a nap* and come back to a fantastic meal! That's good for you, too!

As far as we know, that's about the coolest thing ever. They're meals that *cook themselves* for heaven's sake!

Chapter 4 – But it's a good thing you don't actually have to choose

Let's be realistic here...

You're probably going to have both a pressure cooker and a slow cooker in your kitchen. You should. They're both amazing and unique in their own ways. Both fantastic ways to cook food.

The differences are certainly there, though-- and you'll find that over time you'll have a preference for one over the other. That's okay. That is normal; you're just forming habits at that point and that's a normal thing to do.

With both of these cookers, you'll be able to prepare all kinds of dishes and foods for you and your folks. And you'll be able to eat healthy. In fact, there's a lot that slow cookers and pressure cookers have in common, speaking from a purely academic and culinary standpoint.

So slow cookers and pressure cookers alike are extremely vegetarian friendly. This is good because vegetables are just the better food choice that everyone should have more of. If everyone on the planet could be a vegetarian, we'd probably end world hunger and all kinds of nasty things that we don't want-- so it's good that both of these methods of cooking are veggie-friendly.

Now there are differences in the way these two kitchen implements actually cook food. Of course, the foods and veggies that are cooked in the pressure cooker are going to have more distinct and individual flavors and textures than they would have if they were cooked all together in a slow cooker over night or something.

However, that's a good thing for some people-- but it can of course be viewed as a flavor/texture thing that you're really missing out on if you're partial to cooking with a slow cooker.

Both ways of cooking are extremely efficient. Pressure cookers cook whole meals very quickly though their clever use of high pressure. Slow cookers are very efficient in that they're really practical to use and they don't require you to stand over your food while it's being cooked-- thereby meaning that you don't have to spend as much effort cooking a meal if you're using a slow cooker.

But sometimes you're not out to be as lazy as possible; sometimes you want to actually spend that thirty or so minutes in the kitchen just making food; that's part of the process.

Both pressure cookers and slow cookers alike are very flexible with the number of servings that you're cooking. So you can cook for yourself, or you can cook for many people at a time with both and the cooking process is pretty much the same.

Though, there is one benefit that a slow cooker has over a pressure cooker on that front. The slow cooker's food is more freezer-friendly. Those homogeneously blended food items and stews can be frozen, stored, and thawed later and still maintain their tastiness.

In contrast, the pressure cooker's foods tend to need you to put them in specialized freezer bags in order for them to retain their taste and texture. This is all different from the other cooker in this regard. But some people don't actually ever freeze and store their food-- so if you're one of these people with a more or less empty freezer all the time, this advantage that a slow cooker has over a pressure cooker might not really score any points for you.

So keep that in mind if you're prone to make a bunch of food and store it for a long time to enjoy later once you re-heat it.

But then again, if you're making food to freeze it and re-heat it later, aren't you basically going through the trouble of cooking the same meal twice but only enjoying it once? In a lot of senses, thawing is actually as slow or slower than pressure cooking is since pressure cooking is so amazingly fast and satisfying to begin with. So weigh your options carefully... or not so carefully... since like... nothing's really at stake here. Just your consideration.

Aside from that, you can cook meat with both of these methods. And both times, the proteins and fats that are included in meats are stored in the food and are able to be consumed for their whole nutritional value. So you can enjoy that with both methods of food prep. You can cook more than just vegetarian meals with them. You can even cook really exotic meats and dishes like lamb or swordfish and the dish will still come out awesome!

The aromas that are produced by both methods of cooking (sense the sense of smell is part of the sensation of the full dining experience) are amazing as well. They will both often fill your house with unique and food-like aromas that whet the appetite. Though the smells are somewhat distinct from one another. You can sometimes tell what's been slow-cooking for a while versus what's been cooked in a pressure cooker. Slow-cooker scents and aromas tend to linger and fill a house for a longer time than pressure-cooker aromas. It's just a characteristic of the cooking methods.

Though some people say that pressure cookers carry sweeter-smelling food-aromas with them, and slow cookers tend to give earthy-smells-- this is somewhat debated by food-lovers.

Either way. Odds are, you're not really going to have to settle for one over the other; both of these cookers can be bought just about anywhere for relatively inexpensive prices.

The name brands that you can get with slow cookers and pressure cookers aren't really of major importance here-- you can expect to pay about fifty bucks for a good pressure cooker and about thirty or fifty dollars for a good slow cooker. Of course, the prices and name-brands go up from there and all that; but it's really more about finding what suits your needs.

Any brand is relatively sufficient for starters, though you might want to move into your higher-up name brands like pampered chef once you get really serious about what recipes you like and what your personal cooking niche truly is. But don't really fret too much over name brands and where you can get the very-very best for the very-very lowest price; generally you're only talking about a difference of ten or so dollars when you're comparing similar-qualities in your kitchen utensils.

So don't settle! Try them both! We recommend getting two inexpensive cookers; one of each, and trying each of them out to see what you like the most. If you like one particular thing, then you can graduate to a more expensive brand from there with that.

Either way, there's really no way to go wrong.

Conclusion

The conclusion is that there really is no definitive conclusion. Personally, I like my slow cooker more than I like my pressure cooker. I enjoy being able to spend relatively ten minutes of my time making a dinner for five on my "whatever" ingredients and satisfying my whole family with that on just a few dollars of ingredients.

My mother enjoys a good pressure cooker though. She enjoys being able to cook a good meal in under an hour with the 'real-food' taste and flavors that come with cooking from home. I cannot blame her; she is, after all, a more experienced cook than I am.

However, you may find yourself in a similar situation of not having a very strong preference either way but having both and understanding the advantages and disadvantages that come with either style of cooking.

Or you might find yourself to be a die-hard fan of one style of cooking and vehemently insisting that you'll *never* use the other method of cooking. That's fine too; there are no wrong answers here. Just costs and benefits.

You'll find that the more you cook with both of these in your house, the more you'll tend to favor using one over the other, and the firmer your habits and cooking styles will be. I'd recommend really trying both for a solid month or so before deciding whether to chuck your pressure cooker or your slow cooker in favor for the other one that you decided to keep and love forever.

You can't really go wrong with either one. They're both very good choices for being efficient in the kitchen-- though they're both efficient in very different ways, respectively-- and they open up a wide range of food options for healthy living that previously wasn't there before for most people who choose to cook at home.

The home economics of using these kinds of cookers is phenomenal as well; in the case of the slow cooker it almost really is "stone soup for dinner!" but slow cookers are much more... traditional... in ways. It feels more like *cooking* than slow cookers do.

Slow cookers feel like brewing more than cooking.

But don't be too caught up in the debate. Just understand the costs and benefits of both styles and go from there. There are no wrong answers!